Sutcliffe —   B

ARTHRITIS

A naturopathic practitioner examines the
many causes of arthritis and provides a
programme of natural self-help remedies to
combat this all-too-common condition.

D1332864

ARTHRITIS

EXAMINES THE CAUSES
AND SELF-TREATMENT OF
THIS PAINFUL CONDITION USING
NATURAL HEALING METHODS

LEON CHAITOW
N.D., D.O.

Thorsons
An Imprint of HarperCollins*Publishers*

Thorsons
An Imprint of HarperCollins*Publishers*
77–85 Fulham Palace Road,
Hammersmith, London W6 8JB.

Published by Thorsons 1987
9 10 8

© Thorsons Publishing Group 1987

Leon Chaitow asserts the moral right to
be identified as the author of this work

British Library Cataloguing in Publication Data

Chaitow, Leon
Arthritis. – (The New self-help series)
1. Arthritis – Treatment 2. Rheumatism
– Treatment 3. Self-care. Health
I. Title II. Series
616.07′2068   RC933

ISBN 0-7225-1416-6

Printed in Great Britain by
HarperCollins Manufacturing, Glasgow

Contents

Note to reader

Introduction

Most people, by the time they are middle aged (say forty upwards), will have some degree of osteoarthritis in their body. The most likely sites are in the weight-bearing joints of the body, hips, knees, spine, etc. In many cases the only sign of the condition will be a degree of stiffness, and seldom much pain. Pain however will become evident if these compromised joints are asked to perform tasks which are no longer easy for them.

Man has been described as a two-legged creature with a backache. The backache suffered by most middle aged people relates to some degree of osteoarthritis and the reasons for the human animal's back problems are thought to relate to a failure to adapt fully to the upright position.

In evolutionary terms the way the spine was carried when, in distant history, man's forebears were on all fours, provided the spinal structures with adequate support and shock absorbing capacity. A leading spinal researcher, Professor Korr of Texas University School of Osteopathic Medicine, has noted the change thus: 'The spine of man is a perfect cantilever bridge (when in the all-fours position) and has been turned through a 90 degree angle and is now an unstable skyscraper'. We are apparently faced with nature's uncompleted adaptation as a cause of our weak backs. This is a major reason for the development of osteoarthritis, as the stresses and strains of use in modern life impose their wear and tear on the joints of this region.

Failure to adapt to other aspects of life, nutritional in the main, may well lie behind some cases of rheumatoid arthritis, which has elements in its make up of allergy and self-allergy (autoimmune disease). In many cases this has been shown to be the result of a combination of nutrient deficiency and intolerance to certain foods, notably those which have been introduced to man's diet in comparitively recent history, such as grains and dairy produce.

Some of the strategies available to us in dealing with these problems, in a self-help manner, are explained in later chapters. They are not always easy answers though, and in some cases the best that can be hoped for is a coping strategy rather than cure, since once joint surfaces are damaged beyond a certain point they cannot be expected to regenerate. Safe pain-relief, improvement of mobility and reduction of inflammatory processes are the major elements in self-help methods. These entail both externally and internally applied measures involving nutrients and herbal substances.

Medical care is largely palliative in these conditions. Most of the drugs used in rheumatology are dangerous, some extremely so, including cortisone and the common anti-inflammatory drugs (Butizolidin, Opren, etc) which have been discredited because of the widespread deaths they have caused and have now been withdrawn from the market. Surgery offers a chance of a new lease of life in many cases of joint destruction, and the technical brilliance of these operations should be applauded, even if they are patching up damage rather than curing it. Such methods are most successful in hips and knees, and to large extent finger joints damaged beyond repair by arthritic processes, but are no answer to multiple joint problems.

Prevention must remain the major objective, and this is best achieved by a balanced diet, good body use and the ability to cope well with stress factors. Attention to the overall use of the body in work, home and play, in terms of minimizing stresses and strains on the mechanical component generally and the spine in particular is most important in this respect. Advice and attention from a qualified osteopathic or chiropractic practitioner, on the basis of check-ups every six months, even if there are no problems, is a wise precaution to take, and should be adopted for children from their early years. In this manner much mechanical damage can be avoided and much suffering prevented.

In the following chapters we will be examining the major areas of arthritic change, osteoarthritis and rheumatoid arthritis. There are many other conditions which can loosely be grouped together as arthritic or rheumatic, but these two major areas are the ones we will concentrate upon. The self-help measures outlined can well be adapted to most joint problems however, since they are not harmful if performed in the manner advised.

Self-help involves effort and continuity. Few of the measures mentioned will do much if performed only once or twice, or if not continued over a long period. This is especially true of nutritional methods which are literally trying to alter the biochemistry of the body. This is seldom achieved speedily, and should be viewed as an on-going pattern if relief is found to chronic problems.

All healing comes from within and the measures in this book attempt to deal with all aspects of man, physical and mental, to offer the processes and ingredients which can allow healing to the extent possible in any case and to provide relief where healing is not fully possible.

1.

What is Arthritis?

Before arthritic sufferers can help themselves recover from, or control, arthritis it is useful for them to understand that term. All animals which have a back bone, including man, are prone to arthritis and apparently have been throughout history. Evidence of this condition can be found in prehistoric man and also in the skeletons of the dinosaurs.

Osteoarthritis is a condition rather than a disease and it can have a variety of causes. Rheumatoid arthritis however is a disease and both it and osteoarthritis are not in any way related except that in the late stages of rheumatoid arthritis, when the active inflammation of the joints is 'burned-out', some osteoarthritic changes develop. The need to clarify just which type of arthritis is present will become apparent when we understand just how different the two types are from one another. There is of course a large number of conditions which carry the label 'arthritis', but in the main these are rare, so it is our task to describe some of the causes of osteoarthritis and rheumatoid arthritis, and then to give suggestions as to how self-help methods can be applied.

All arthritic changes affecting joints can be described as degenerative joint diseases, or conditions. The causes lie in a variety of factors including heredity, ageing, wear and tear, posture, occupation, nutrition, allergies, injury, infection, body weight, inflammatory factors, and hormonal alterations or they may be any combination of these, and other, factors.

Osteoarthritis is that form of arthritis which is most responsible for incapacity, loss of time from work, and general disability. It affects mainly the hips, knees, spine and fingers (fingers and knees are more affected in women, and hips and the spine in men). Bearing in mind that we are discussing different and distinct conditions, and that the word arthritis can be applied to quite separate entities, we will begin by examining osteoarthritis, the all-pervasive form.

Osteoarthritis can manifest itself as early as the late teens, and is probably present (although usually with few or no symptoms) in nearly everyone by the time they are in their seventies. It is a local condition which means that its development is not usually accompanied by systemic changes in the blood or in the body as a whole. It appears in one or several joints co-incidentally. Obviously if the state of the individual's body is such as to allow the development of degenerative changes in one joint, it will be the same for any other joints that may be similarly under postural, mechanical or traumatic stress. What actually takes place in a joint which is becoming osteoarthritic is a wearing away of the smooth, polished cartilage, which is the gliding interface lying between the bones of a joint. This wearing process tends to expose the underlying bone to wear and pressure. Particles of damaged cartilage and bone become irritated and ultimately inflamed as a result and there is a protective effort on the part of the body to repair, splint, or cushion the damaged area. This involves enzymes, blood cells, etc, and regardless of the initial cause or the actual body response, the underlying cartilage, and the fluid in which it is bathed, begin to show signs of change. There is an attempt to reinforce the damaged cartilage structure, and fluid from the joint may be unable to sustain its nutritive role, which is to help maintain and regenerate the cartilage. This failure to maintain the cartilage may take place during a major inflammatory stage, or through repetitive overuse, associated with minor inflammation of the area. As the cartilage develops increasing signs of wear, and the underlying bone becomes irritated, there is a proliferation of the bone as new cells are laid down to deal with the injury. The new bone forms outcroppings known as osteophytes, and these grow larger as the cartilage becomes increasingly worn away. By this stage the structure and shape of the end of the bone will have begun to alter and there will be alterations too in the degree and range of free movement in the joint.

This more restricted movement may result in greater stress as the individual attempts to use a severely affected joint. There are therefore waves of inflammation, each of which further aggravates the wear and tear process, with consequent desperate local attempts by the body to splint and rebuild the damaged joint surface. This results in the vicious cycle of damage and pain repeating itself over again. Once movement has been severely compromised the repetition of this cycle declines, because effectively the body will have prevented movement and use. By this stage lumpy, deformed joints are often evident. These are frequently unstable, but may be relatively painless, unless attempts to use them are made. This represents a typical development of an osteoarthritic joint. It may take months or even years for such a joint to reach a stable, but almost totally damaged, state.

It may however never deteriorate to such an extent; instead changes may be minor and the limitations in the movement of the joint remain virtually unnoticed. For example, X-rays of most adults over forty will show some osteoarthritic changes in their necks. However most of these individuals will be completely symptom free. It may therefore be assumed that the process of repair and new bone growth, which the body institutes in response to wear of the joint surface, is nearly always successfully achieved.

That is to say that this form of arthritis is often actually helpful, in that it protects the damaged joint surface from greater destruction. It is only when this process is accompanied by excessive inflammation, and repeated laying down of new bone growth, that extreme limitation occurs. Thus the factors which need to be examined are those that determine the degree of inflammation, and the ability of the body to respond adequately, without going beyond what is desirable in the way of repair and splinting.

If most people have pain-free joints which show signs of osteoarthritis, it must be assumed that this is part of the marvellous self-maintenance mechanism of the body. After all, the body would cease to function adequately if it did not attempt to repair the initial stages of cartilage wear for then the cartilage would simply wear away and the bone underlying it would do the same. The response of the body has to be sufficient to protect the underlying bone so that further damage is avoided and joint movement is not impeded. If osteoarthritis is tackled at an early stage and the body is assisted in the task of repair, then there is every chance that the amount of damage can be contained, and a virtually symptomless stage reached. For this to happen the underlying causes need to be found and then rectified. This may entail losing weight, improving posture, or reducing habitual or occupational stress. It also entails providing the body generally, and the joint specifically with the optimum environment for repair. This means that the nutritional status of the individual must be at its optimum so that the nutrients vital for repair are present. It also means that local circulation and muscle tone must be at their best as both are necessary for repair and maintenance of joints. This calls for a variety of exercises to improve muscle tone and enhance circulation efficiency. By removing the underlying causes, helping the repair process, enhancing the efficiency of circulation, and improving muscle tone most osteoarthritic conditions will be improved, and often become symptom free. (This is provided that the damage of joints has not advanced beyond a point of no return.)

Even if damage has progressed beyond such a stage, however, there is still much that can be done firstly to prevent the progression of the condition, and then hopefully to reduce pain, stiffness and associated disability as much as possible. The self-help methods that we will be discussing in subsequent chapters are ones which can easily be applied at home. Of course there are specialized treatments which do not fall within the scope of self-help. These include the use of osteopathic and chiropractic manipulation to help normalize body mechanics; acupuncture to relieve pain and stiffness and enhance circulation; physiotherapy, including ultrasonic therapy, to help localized inflammation to be contained; surgical measures to actually replace damaged joints; and splinting and support for damaged joints, such as the knee, which may have become unstable. Such measures, although lying beyond the scope of this book, should be borne in mind. But a note of caution should be added; the standard medical therapy for osteoarthritis, involving the use of anti-inflammatory drugs, has been shown to cause much suffering, and even death. Many anti-arthritic drugs which have arrived in a blaze of publicity have been withdrawn after a few years under a cloud of suspicion that they involve far more suffering than ever they relieved. Aspirin is still the safest of all anti-arthritic drugs, for all its shortcomings.

The methods we will be discussing do not involve drugs. Should the individual be taking drugs, under medical supervision, there is no reason whatever why the methods outlined here should not be employed, for they are supportive of the body and have no bad side effects. Having found a programme which helps to minimize the causes of the condition, and which enhances the defensive ability of the body, it may well be that drugs can be phased out. Self-help is the aim; this does of course call for some application and effort on the patient's part. Intelligent cooperation in any programme is essential. It is not advisable to undertake diets and exercises grudgingly or half-heartedly. Rather, see the good sense of what is involved and plunge in with a good heart, with the long term view of better health, greater mobility and the use of presently compromised joints. This is the way to begin helping the body to recover.

Before looking at any of the individual

methods that will help the body we must consider the other major arthritic condition, namely rheumatoid arthritis. This is a chronic, usually progressive inflammatory disorder of the joints. It is more common in women than men and occurs at any age, but usually between the ages of twenty-five and fifty-five. The condition usually involves bilateral symptoms, that is, it occurs on both sides of the body at the same time. Very occasionally it may appear on one side only, and if so it usually involves the knees. The symmetrical, two-sided development of symptoms is distinctive of rheumatoid arthritis, since osteoarthritis usually affects only one joint. The inflammatory process in rheumatoid arthritis is usually progressive and, depending upon the severity of the attack, can completely destroy the joints' ability to function, leaving them swollen and distorted. The affected joints will also be warm or even hot, reddened and tender, at least during the active phase of the disease. There is a characteristic stiffness in the mornings, which tends to last half an hour or so, but which may last for hours. At the outset it is the pain which limits movement, but as time passes the supporting tissues of the joints change and fibrosis occurs which limits the elasticity of the area.

Limitation of movement may become profound and ankylosis may occur. This means that bones which normally have a degree of movement between them actually become fused. Initially, the joints most commonly affected are those of the hands, feet, wrists and knees. Later this may spread to the elbows, shoulders, ankles, hips and collar bone. Sometimes the jaw may become affected. In rheumatoid arthritis the spine is rarely affected, unlike osteoarthritis. Should it be it usually only involves the neck region.

In the fingers, early signs of rheumatoid arthritis are manifest in joints which swell and become spindle-shaped. This often clears after a few years as the condition progresses to other areas. There is often a deformity of the fingers so that there is a twisting outwards of the joints to produce a deviation from the normal position. This is combined with damage to the tendons which guide the joints. This may result in distortion producing abnormal flexion of the fingers so that it becomes impossible to bring the finger tips together. This makes the lifting of small objects very difficult and sometimes impossible. Such distortion is possible in any affected joint, and the disability and progressive pain which this produces makes it a nightmare of endurance.

The onset is frequently accompanied by loss of weight and appetite, fatigue and unaccountable fever and sweats. There may be obvious nodules, which can be felt under the skin, and there is often generalized aching and stiffness, not at first localized to the joints themselves. At first, the sufferer may only be aware of the involvement of the joints. However, many other systemic changes may occur, including inflammation of the blood vessels, weakness and wasting of muscles, inflammation of the heart muscle (in about 40% of cases). Breathing and sometimes eyes may be affected and lymph glands and spleen may become swollen. Anaemia usually accompanies this disease, despite the fact that the body is not short of iron. It seems that there is an inability to utilize the iron supply adequately. The disease is systemic, in that the whole organism is involved, and this makes it different from osteoarthritis in which only specific joints are affected.

The causes of rheumatoid arthritis are unknown, although the processes that occur are minutely understood. The major theory suggests that rheumatoid arthritis is due to an unnatural behaviour of the body's immune system, so that, for reasons which are unclear, the defence mechanisms actually attack the body tissues, in this case articular joint tissues. Thus, the very elements which are designed to protect the body attack it. Why this should happen is uncertain, but it seems probable that a number of factors must be present simultaneously to account for it. The 'unorthodox' theories regarding the cause of this disease will be discussed later.

Statistics confirm that, of any one hundred rheumatoid arthritis sufferers, fifteen will have only a short-lived disease (which will remit of its own accord, with no treatment, and leave very little permanent damage). A further twenty-five will have episodes which persist for some time, (perhaps months or even years) but will also remit, leaving few after-effects, apart from slight joint distortion and a little stiffness. A further fifty will have persistent symptoms. They will suffer periods of distress interspersed with periods of remission, gradually leading to deformity and varying degrees of disability. The remaining ten will suffer the relentless progression of the disease, usually quite unresponsive to any treatment, and leading to complications and probable wheelchair confinement.

If remission is going to occur spontaneously, then this usually takes place in the first year, especially if the disease had an acute onset. In general, men have a better chance of remission than women, especially if the disease begins before the age of forty-five. If there are manifestations of rheumatoid arthritis in areas other than the joints, the prognosis is less good. This is also true if there is X-ray evidence of erosion of the bone surface in affected joints.

The signs that identify rheumatoid arthritis include the following: stiffness in the mornings, with pain on movement in at least one joint; swelling of at least one joint, and more probably of the same joint on both sides of the body; and nodules, which can be felt over prominent bones, or near joints. Apart from these signs there are distinctive bone changes, visible on X-ray, showing inflammation as well as detectable changes in the blood. The greater the number of symptoms which are manifest, the greater the chances that the condition is rheumatoid arthritis. (The above symptoms must be present for at least six weeks continuously. Shorter periods are probably not the result of rheumatoid arthritis.)

The self-help programme designed to alleviate the symptoms, and improve the general health of the sufferer, will be described later. Some of the advice is applicable to both rheumatoid arthritis and osteoarthritis, for instance, in both cases an inflamed joint can be helped by hydrotherapy. On the other hand, this is not always the case and specific advice for rheumatoid arthritic conditions will also be given.

In order to cope with a problem which manifestly involves all aspects of the body it is necessary to advise a reform of the whole pattern of life. This must include adequate rest and exercise, nutritional reform, specific supplementation, psychological reorientation and guided imagery, hydrotherapy and the use of helpful herbal and other non-toxic sub-stances.

One area which needs careful evaluation is that of allergy. It has been demonstrated that some rheumatoid patients are in fact displaying a marked reaction against particular foods, and that when these are removed from the diet a dramatic improvement is possible. This is not by any means always the case, but it is desirable to reassess the food that one eats as it relates to the chemical additives which enter the body. Thus, a key aspect of a self-help programme is the detoxification of the body which effectively rids the system of any toxic encumberances which may contribute to rheumatoid arthritis. For instance, this involves the use of methods which ensures a regular bowel function. Other methods will be discussed in subsequent chapters. Some experts have suggested that the combination of allergic reactions to foods and chemical and toxic factors, may be the ultimate cause of the faulty immune reaction in which the body attacks itself.

A large number of other so-called rheumatoid or arthritic conditions exist, which are not dealt with in this book. These include gout, and all the soft tissue conditions so often lumped together as 'fibrocitis and rheumatism'. These will be dealt with in another book in this series titled 'Rheumatic Ailments'. There is an overlap between all these conditions, and some of the advice is applicable to several of them. For instance, in all cases the detoxification of the body and the removal of stress are important factors and greatly contribute to the body's self-healing ability.

2.

The Causes of Osteoarthritis

The way we use our body, day in and day out, greatly affects its wear and tear. Posture and habitual use determine the degree of repetitive strain imposed upon joints. Habits of use generally begin in infancy, and so are not particularly easy to correct in adult life. The human spine has been aptly described as a superb cantilever bridge which has been inadequately adapted for use as a skyscraper. The main factor which constantly produces strain on the body, and the spine in particular, is gravity. If the spine is not correctly balanced, strains are imposed upon certain of the articulating surfaces.

If we consider the other everyday strains which are added to the stresses caused by poor posture, then we can appreciate the great number of strains to which our bodies are subject. Footwear is a major cause of strain. High heels, especially, throw the weight of the body forward of its centre of gravity. This results in alterations in muscular patterns which in turn place increased weight on joints which were never designed for such stresses. The hips, knees, feet and joints of the lower back and pelvis are particularly involved in such strains.

The regular use of poorly designed furniture is another factor in unnatural wear and tear. Chairs which provide inadequate support, or which are too low or too high, in relation to body size and particular activities (e.g., typing), contribute to body strain. Newer designs of chairs, from Scandinavia, allow for a degree of kneeling, and consequently provide a far more desirable spinal contour than traditional chairs. Such chairs are now increasingly becoming available from specialist 'back shops', and the better of the office supply companies.

Beds that are too soft, work surfaces that are the wrong height, or working conditions which impose undesirable stresses, contribute further to repetitive muscular and joint strains. In addition, weight bearing joints are exposed to undue stress if the body weight is above normal, and also if weight carrying or lifting is a regular feature of daily life.

Given that the above factors contribute significantly to osteoarthritic problems, they need to be carefully considered. Is there a degree of overweight? Are there repetitive daily habits which might be unduly straining joints and muscles? Are there habits of posture related to occupation (e.g., typing, hairdressing, lifting) which cause stress? Are there repetitive activities (e.g., sport or hobbies) which might be adding to the strain of joints? Is posture satisfactory? What changes can be made to reduce the stresses that might result from any of the above?

Less obvious factors might be considered. Sitting with legs crossed is a common cause of undue lower back and hip joint torsion and strain; standing habitually with the body weight on one leg is another. Both may result from a pelvic or spinal imbalance which in turn has resulted in one leg appearing to be longer than the other. This should be assessed and dealt with by a qualified osteopathic or chiropractic practitioner. Habits which favour one side of the body should be eliminated. One such habit is the tucking of a telephone between the ear and the shoulder. If this is a common habit, it may result in strain on the neck region with consequent aggravation of arthritic changes, which are all too common in that area.

Observation of our daily habits can help us evaluate those which are unduly stressful and we can begin to eliminate them. For instance, loss of surplus weight is beneficial, and dealing with apparent or real imbalances, such as short-leg problems, is also useful. Frequently, however, osteoarthritic changes may well be established by the time we become aware of such factors, and changes in lifestyle may not eliminate the problems. Yet they can be important in reducing pain and discomfort, and in slowing or checking progression of the condition. It may be useful to look at ourselves in photographs, so as to check for habitual tilting of the head, or other obvious postural imbalances. Look to see whether eyes, ears, and shoulders are level. Such factors provide clues to deviations in the contour of the spine, and these deviations may benefit from regular stretching exercises, as well as from attention by a practitioner skilled in spine and body mechanics.

Long before joint problems become manifest there will have been a tendency for the soft tissues of the region to become stiffer and tighter than usual. Often this is taken simply as part of the ageing process and so is endured. Yet, were attention paid to early stiffness in muscles and soft tissues, there is a good chance that the insidious onset of joint dysfunction and ultimate osteoarthritic change might have been prevented. It is important that after any injury (such as a fall, jar or blow) that leaves a region less than fully free and mobile, attention should be given by a suitably qualified practitioner. Sporting injuries often become arthritic many years later, simply as a result of inadequate attention at the time of injury. Motor car accidents, especially those involving violent jarring (such as whiplash of the neck) can have similar long term effects. If the soft tissues are given attention soon after such injuries, then joint damage is more likely to be avoided.

Emotional strain, which produces a tensing and contracting of groups of muscles, is another cause of osteoarthritic changes. It can impair joint movement and circulation. Such effects of

emotional stress may be overcome by regular
stretching exercises, such as those used in yoga,
as well as stress reduction methods. These
methods are discussed in the following chapter.

3.

Self-help Therapy

Stretching exercises

The following stretching exercises are recommended as part of a general prevention programme. They may not be entirely suitable for all arthritic sufferers. If they hurt then they are being done too enthusiastically, and require modification. If they do not hurt during performance, and leave the area more supple, then they are desirable. Specific exercises can be used for specific areas, however the following are meant for general stretching and limbering. They are appropriate for individuals with osteoarthritis, rheumatoid arthritis or stiffness, as long as *no pain results*.

These exercises are meant to produce general effects. To start with do the following movements three times each. After a few days increase them to ten times each.

Stand up straight with your feet apart and your hands clasped behind your back. Allow yourself to bend forward from the hips as far as is comfortable. Use no effort but try to allow the weight of the upper body to stretch you forwards. Feel the stretch up the back of your legs and especially behind the knees. This exercise is not repeated. You simply hold the position for half a minute; breathe slowly and deeply, and allow the stretch to reach its maximum. As the days go by allow the time in this position to increase to three minutes. This stretches the hamstrings, helps the muscular supporting structures of the pelvis, and improves abdominal tone, but it is important to breathe slowly and deeply all the while.

For the following exercise you may, at first, need to hold onto a solid object, such as heavy table, in order not to lose your balance. If you can do it unaided, so much the better. With feet about 12–15 inches (30–38 cm) apart and standing up straight, slowly go into a squatting position, trying to keep your heels on the floor. If this is not possible then either go just as far as you can into the squat without raising your heels, or wear high heels when doing the exercise. As you squat, stretch your arms forward and lean forward from the waist to maintain balance. If you feel you are toppling backwards you may need to balance yourself by holding onto a table or some other heavy object. When you are at the fullest limit of your squat give a few gentle up and down 'jigs' as though you are trying to tuck your tail between your legs. Rise and repeat.

This exercise tones the hamstrings, acts as a

general stimulant to circulation and muscle tone in the pelvic area, and stretches the lower back. When it becomes easy to perform you can vary it by using the more advanced technique of interlocking the fingers behind the neck as you start (head facing straight ahead). At the end of each deep squat rise to your feet slowly, and as you do so stretch the hands (still interlocked) towards the ceiling, pressing open palms as far upwards as possible. This is further enhanced by breathing in deeply as you stretch upwards. Repeat three to ten times.

The following variations on chair exercises are designed to achieve general stretching of the upper part of the body, without strain. First, sit on an ordinary dining chair, feet together and hands clasped behind the back. Bend forward from the waist with the hands stretching backwards and upwards as far as possible. Your trunk should be leaning as far forward as possible, so that your nose is as close to your knees as it can get. The hands should stretch up and back and be held there for five to ten seconds, as you breathe in and out. Sit up and repeat.

After doing this a number of times separate your feet so that there is a wide gap between your knees. Repeat the exercise, but instead of bending straight forwards, bend towards each knee alternately. This time keep the hands clasped behind the back without stretching them backwards. Repeat several times in each direction, holding for a full cycle of breathing.

Sit straight up in the chair, feet together and

arms extended sideways, palms downwards. Breathe in and turn the palms upwards and at the same time stretch the arms backwards so that you feel the shoulder blades coming towards each other. Relax and breathe out as you let the arms resume their original position. Repeat.

Sitting, place your hands behind your neck, or rest the fingertips on the shoulders, whichever is the more comfortable. Slowly rotate the shoulders so that your arms are moving in a gentle circle (as though you are drawing circles with your elbows). Repeat in each direction several times. You should try to achieve maximum stretch as the elbows circle, so that they go back, then down, then forward, then up as far as possible in each direction of circling.

Relaxation

This method of relaxation should be introduced at the outset of any self-help approach to healing. Whilst learning the technique, arrange to have two free periods per day, each of five to fifteen minutes duration. Find a quiet room where you know you will not be disturbed. Rest on your back, with head and shoulders slightly raised, and pillows under the knees to take the strain off them and your back. Rest your hands on the upper abdomen, close your eyes, settle down in a comfortable position. Ensure that there is nothing to distract your attention, such as sunlight, a clock, or animals. Sitting in a reclining position is also suitable, and many people prefer this to lying down. Try both, and choose whichever is most comfortable.

Breathing is of great value in relaxation, particularly during the initial stages. It is partly carried out through the autonomic nervous system and partly through the central nervous system. The autonomic nervous system is that which controls vital functions, endocrine (hormone) secretions and emotions. By controlling one's breathing, one can influence all these functions and, for a short time, take over conscious responsibility from them. Breathing is the only automatic function which one is easily able to control.

The aim is to breathe slowly, deeply and rhythmically. You cannot expect to do this perfectly from the start — it might take weeks. Inhale through the nose slowly and deeply. The abdomen, on which the hands are resting, should rise gently as the breathing begins. An awareness of this rising and falling of the abdomen is important to establish that the diaphragm is being used properly. Inhalation should be slow, unforced and unhurried. Whilst breathing in, slowly and silently, count to four, five or six. When the inhalation is complete, pause for two or three seconds, then slowly exhale through the nose. As you exhale, you should feel the abdomen slowly falling. While breathing out count again to four, five or six. The exhalation should take at least as long as the inhalation.

There should be no sense of strain when breathing. If at first you feel that you have breathed to your fullest capacity by a count of three, work gradually to improve it. Try to slow down the rhythm until a slow count of five or six is possible, both on inhalation and exhalation, with a pause of two or three seconds in between. Remember to start each breath with an upwards push of the abdomen. With the mind thus occupied on the mechanics of breathing and the rhythmic counting, there is little scope for thinking about anything else. Nevertheless, initially at least, extraneous thoughts will intrude. This pattern of breathing should be repeated fifteen to twenty times and, since each cycle should take about fifteen seconds, this exercise should occupy a total of about five minutes.

Once slow, rhythmic breathing becomes well established it is useful to introduce a pattern of thoughts during different phases of the breathing cycle. For example, on inhalation, try to sense a feeling of warmth and energy entering the body with the air. On exhaling, sense a feeling of sinking and settling deeper into the supporting surface. An overall sense of warmth and heaviness accompanying the repetitive breathing cycle will enhance relaxation. Physiologically, this exercise will slow down the heart rate, reduce sympathetic nervous activity, relax tense muscles and allow a chance for the balancing, restorative, parasympathetic nervous functions to operate. It calms the mind as well.

After a few weeks begin to introduce specific images into your thought patterns of any painful or restricted areas being freed and loosened. 'See' the muscles letting go and feel the circulation coursing through the tissues.

With this image try to see any affected areas as moving and pain free. Spend a minute or so on any joint or area that is a problem. Visualization of this sort has a definite physiological effect and deserves repetition daily.

The use of regular stretching exercises, and of a general relaxation method, is an important first step in getting the body harnassed to the task of recovery. If walking is not a problem then regular walking should also be introduced. At least twenty minutes every other day (more if possible), should be the aim. As an alternative, swimming offers the safest and most beneficial exercise for anyone with either osteoarthritis or rheumatoid arthritis.

Exercise during periods of acute arthritic pain should however, be limited. Slow movements which stretch tight muscles and tone weak ones, painlessly, are highly desirable in such circumstances. The level of activity desirable should be tailored to your particular condition, so it is not possible to be specific here. However, walking or swimming should be brisk enough in general to leave the individual slightly out of breath, but not sufficient to cause any distress or pain. By regular exercise the same distance can be covered in a progressively shorter time, as fitness improves; or better still the distance covered in the time allotted can gradually be increased.

Stretching and relaxation exercises, together with walking or swimming, will improve general circulation, including the flow of lymphatic fluid, which acts as the main channel of detoxification of the body. In this way specific and local changes will take place, despite the general nature of the exercises.

Muscle energy methods

More localized attention can be given to any restricted joint by using modified muscle energy techniques. An osteopathic manoeuvre exists which can be adapted as a self-help method to ease tight and restricted muscles and joints. These exercises are based on the physiological fact that every muscle, or group of muscles, has an opposing or antagonistic muscle, or set of muscles. When one set of muscles is being used, the opposing set is obliged to relax. This means that muscles which have tightened, or become stiff and restricted, may be eased by making the opposing set of muscles work.

The best way of doing this is through isometric exercises. This means that the muscle that is used is made to work, without any actual movement taking place. If a joint is restricted in movement, for instance, if the elbow is difficult to straighten, then it should be gently taken to the comfortable limit, *in the direction in which it is restricted*. This means that an attempt is made to place the arm in the maximum degree of straightness, without causing pain. At that point the other hand is placed on the forearm (which could be resting on the arm of a chair), so as to restrict the next stage of the operation, which is a firm, steady — not jerky — attempt to bend the arm. The restriction placed on the arm by the other hand should *exactly* match the effort being made to bend the arm. Thus, of course, no movement should take place. This effort and counter effort should be maintained for five to ten seconds before a gradual easing of effort is allowed and the arm is rested for a few seconds.

At that point it may be possible, without force or pain, to obtain a little more movement, and the arm may straighten a little more easily. Again the joint should be taken to the limit of the restricted movement and the same procedure adopted as before, with the arm bent, resisted by the counter pressure of the other hand (but not using your full strength). Allow a period of five to ten seconds during which the pressures exactly match each other before releasing the arm. Then test the joint again to see if a little more of its normal range of movement has been reached.

This method can be used on most joints in the body. However, it cannot always be used on joints which are not *easily accessible*, for example, the spinal joints. The joints of the limbs, shoulder and neck, though, are reasonably accessible and so can be adapted to the above exercise. In some cases there is a better result if, while the joint is being thus treated, there is a slow release of the restricting pressure, so as to allow the joint to move, albeit very slowly, in the direction opposite to the main joint restriction.

The number of times that this can be repeated at any one session depends upon the improvement gained. Once the method has been used with no further movement being gained, it is probably all that is required for that joint at that time. Of course, some joints require that the angle at which the restricted movement is attempted be varied, to help develop movement in several different directions. By varying the angle of resisted effort all the muscles of a joint can be brought into play, little by little. At no time should pain be felt when these procedures are being used. Even if no great increase in the range of movement is achieved, perhaps because of existing joint damage, this exercise will still provide relaxation of the soft tissue structures, which in turn will make the area more comfortable.

These types of exercises are of use in either osteoarthritic or rheumatoid conditions, as well as a wide range of muscular rheumatic and fibrocitic states, as long as pain is not precipitated by them. The effort involved should match exactly the comfortable degree of restriction of movement that the free hand or hands can apply.

Trigger point self-treatment
In most arthritic patients there exist specific localized areas, in muscles associated with arthritic joints which, when pressed, are sore both locally and also send pain to another area, sometimes quite a distance away. For example, such points are commonly found in the muscles

between the shoulder and the neck (trapezius muscles). When pressed, these points hurt locally and often send pain and discomfort to the arm, mid-spine or head. Such points are called trigger points because they trigger pain in a target area. They frequently result in the wrong area being treated. For example, a trapezius trigger can cause a more or less constant pain in the side of the neck and head and if these areas are treated no benefit is likely. Only when the trigger is identified and removed, by one means or another, will the pain in the target area disappear.

There are many ways of dealing with such trigger points, including the use of injections. However, the following treatment is one of the best ways of dealing with a trigger point. Firstly, apply pressure by squeezing or directly pressing on the point for about ten seconds. Pressure should be just sufficient to relay discomfort to the target area. After ten seconds ease off for about five seconds and then repeat the pressure. Do this three or four times. Then apply either ice, or a cold spray (obtainable from any pharmacy), to the trigger point, with gentle sweeps towards the target area. The chilling should be done in such a way as to thoroughly cool all the tissues between the trigger and the target, without blanching or frosting the skin. This may take anything from five to twenty seconds, depending on the size of the area involved.

After the chilling, during which time the ice or the spray is kept constantly moving, the muscles should be gently stretched to their comfortable limit. The muscles should be held there for a half a minute or so and then the chilling and stretching should be repeated. This can be done two or three times, after which the trigger point should be less active. This will be apparent in that less discomfort will be felt.

Triggers can be found in any muscle, and are almost always present when a joint has become restricted. Both the 'muscle energy' method, and the chilling and stretching method, will help in keeping such muscles and localized areas from becoming unduly troublesome. Regular treatment of this sort can result in a greatly diminished pain level, and an increased mobility of the joints controlled by muscles thus affected. (More information in identifying and dealing with such points can be found in my book 'Instant Pain Control', Thorsons.)

Hydrotherapy methods

Hydrotherapy can also be used safely to help in rheumatic and arthritic joints. It may have come as a surprise to find that ice was useful in dealing with pain of a rheumatic nature. Usually heat is regarded as soothing and cold as something to be avoided. However it is important to realise that, in certain conditions, cold is infinitely more desirable than heat. The main reason for avoiding cold is that, in some individuals, there is inadequate vitality to respond to such a stimulus. If anyone is febrile, and very weak, then cold applications are best avoided, until the general state of health has improved adequately to respond positively. As a general rule hot applications, or alternate hot and cold applications, are better suited to long standing, chronic conditions. Cold applications are better suited to active inflammatory conditions.

Hydrotherapy can be applied locally or generally, and the following methods are recommended for either osteoarthritis or rheumatoid arthritis.

Cold compress

The cold compress is ideal for all inflamed or stiff joints. Despite its name it is designed to get warm. It is applied cold, but is covered and insulated so as to allow body heat to warm it. A piece of cotton material, large enough to cover the area (wrist, knee, etc) is wrung out in cold tap water, so that it is just damp, but not dripping wet. If the patient is not unduly affected by cold, and has good vitality and circulation, then two thicknesses of material should be used. Patients with poor circulation should settle for one thickness. The compress is placed over the joint and is immediately covered by one or two thicknesses of a flannel or woollen material, which is firmly safety-pinned in place. This is left in position for between four and eight hours, unless it fails to warm up within ten to fifteen minutes. If after this period it still feels cold and clammy, then it was either too damp at the outset or was inadequately insulated. It should be removed and a further attempt made the next day. Normally, it should gradually warm up and will be dry by the time it is removed. It can be left on overnight. The compress has a beneficial effect on the local circulation, as well as on the muscles overlying the joint. It will reduce pain and leave the area feeling easier and more pliable. The cold compress can be used on alternate days. The material used should be well washed after each use, as acid wastes are absorbed via the skin.

Alternate hot and cold bathing

This method is ideal for either acute or chronic joints which are stiff, painful, swollen or inflamed. In order to stimulate the local circulation and reduce swelling and inflamma- tion in an arthritic joint, the use of contrast bathing is ideal. This can be done in a number of ways, depending upon the joints involved. A small joint such as a finger or wrist can be treated under hot and cold running water, or in two bowls with water of appropriate temperatures. The hot water should be of such a temperature as to feel sufficiently hot, but without scalding the skin. The cold water should be very cold. Running tap water is ideal, but if a bowl is used, ice should be floated in the cold water to maintain the temperature. The timing of the alternations is important. The hot treatment should last not less than ten seconds, and the cold not less than five seconds, alternating ten to fifteen times, and finishing with a cold treatment. If a joint (e.g., hip) is not suitable for either of the methods mentioned then towels should be dipped in hot or cold water, lightly wrung out, and then placed over, or round, the affected area. The timing is much the same, so that the towel remains in position for just long enough to prepare the contrasting one. It is a good idea to gently move and stretch the affected joint during and after the hydrotherapy treatment.

Epsom salt bathing

This method is ideal for rheumatic-arthritic conditions and can be used for the whole body, or a local joint. However it is more suitable for chronic stiff conditions rather than acute inflamed ones. If whole body epsom salt bathing is undertaken the patient must be of reasonably sound disposition, as it is a little energy-draining. It is a marvellous method for helping to eliminate toxic wastes via the skin, and is very relaxing. Place, in a normal bath, approximately $2\frac{1}{2}$lbs of commercial epsom salt (available from any chemist). $\frac{1}{2}$lb of common salt (ideally sea salt) and a dessertspoon of iodine. The bath should be at a temperature of 100-104°F/37.7-40°C and the patient should spend between ten and twenty minutes immersed in the water, which should be periodically topped up to maintain the heat. After the bath the patient should be briskly rubbed down, placed in a warm bed and well covered. Normally perspiration is induced by the bath, even in individuals who perspire infrequently. The patient should be given some hours to regain a normal body temperature before venturing out of bed. The epsom salt bath should be not used more than once a week, as it is tiring.

A local joint can be treated in a similar fashion, by soaking it in hot water containing epsom salt, salt and iodine. A hand, foot or elbow can be rested in hot water of this sort for five to ten minutes, and then wrapped in flannel after gentle stretching exercises. The area can be moved and stretched during the bathing as well as afterwards. If an area is too large to 'dunk' in this way, then a towel soaked in the water and wrung out to be just damp can be placed over the area. This should be replaced at frequent intervals to maintain the heat.

General exercise in water

As mentioned in the discussion on general exercise, swimming offers the opportunity to move and stretch joints in a weight-free environment. There is a number of heated pools available in most centres of population. Some are attached to hospitals, some are private and some belong to local authorities. In an uncrowded, heated pool, it should be possible to undertake regular exercise and thereby tone weak muscles, stretch tight joints, and lessen the aggravation of sensitive inflamed tissues. Information regarding hydrotherapy facilities can be obtained from local health authorities, or Citizens Advice Bureaux.

Cryotherapy

As mentioned in the section dealing with trigger points, it is possible to use ice or cold sprays on inflamed areas to advantage. This should be done in such a way as to avoid frosting the skin, or causing any deep cold ache. By chilling the tissues over and around a joint, and then stretching the tissues by slow movement, improved movement can be achieved and pain reduced. If the patient's vitality and circulation are very poor these methods may not be advisable.

There are many other methods of hydro-therapy, but the above are the safest and most desirable for the rheumatic-arthritic conditions under consideration.

Self massage method

The use of gentle massage to assist circulatory efficiency and to reduce congestion and inflammation is very useful. A light lubricant cream or oil should be applied to the area involved, and the muscles and soft tissues should be lightly stroked in the direction of the heart. Pressure can be applied by finger tips, thumb or heel of the hand, in order to drain and 'milk' the area of excess fluid. Use of hydrotherapy after a few minutes of this is particularly desirable. If pressure is hard to apply (and it *is* too hard if it causes pain) then a tennis ball can be used instead. Place the ball over the area involved, and apply pressure to it by rolling it rhythmically onto and across the tight, congested tissues (never enough to hurt). A significant degree of massage will thereby be effected. It is possible to place the ball on the floor, rest the affected part of the body on it, and then gently move the body so as to vary the pressure from the ball on to the affected soft tissues. This is particularly effective in the regions along the spine, and also in the muscles of the lower back, pelvis and hip.

A firm squash-ball can similarly be used on smaller areas such as the forearm. If placed on the forearm, the other hand can gently press the ball into the muscles and roll it about. This can result in a feeling sometimes described as 'nice hurt', since the degree of pressure is under the patient's control. The ball can also be used under the arches of the foot. By resting the foot on the ball, and rolling the foot to and fro, a degree of upward pressure on the arch is achieved. (Greater pressure will be gained by using a golf ball.) Very light pressure achieves marked stretching of the fascia and muscles under the foot. A squash ball can also be used to exercise the hands and fingers. By gently squeezing it between the fingers a variety of muscles can be brought into play, and thus gently assist in the maintenance of strength and movement in affected joints.

Skin friction methods

The skin is a remarkable organ of elimination and we can greatly assist it in this function by regular use of skin friction methods. These are of value to all forms of rheumatic condition as long as they are carried out regularly and not too violently. Not only do they accelerate the removal of wastes from the skin, but they also enhance the lymphatic drainage of the body tissues. The lymphatic system is a waste disposal system, via which a good deal of the breakdown products of life in the cells is carried away for ultimate detoxification and elimination from the body. With age and inactivity these channels become clogged to a large extent. This is especially true of anyone who is less active than usual because of arthritic changes. Skin friction or skin brushing has a remarkable effect on the lymphatic flow helping to reduce swelling in joints. The methods have been in use for many years and are a major part of the revitalizing processes employed by leading health hydros.

The method could not be simpler and involves the use of a brush made with natural (not plastic) bristles, a glove made of hemp or a loofah. Most major chemist chains will stock one or other of these. The brush, glove or loofah is kept dry and the best time for carrying out the (almost) daily ritual is first thing in the morning.

As much of the body surface as is reachable should be brushed (apart from the face). Start if possible with the skin on the feet, both underneath and on the top, then with light strokes at first sweep up the legs, front and back, to the buttocks and hips. The degree of firmness depends upon sensitivity; with regular use this will become greater but at first it will be light. When the abdomen is reached the strokes should be gentle as the skin is much more sensitive, and the pattern should be in a circular motion, going from the top right side of the abdomen across to the left, down and across to the right and then up again to the starting point. This clockwise motion follows the pattern of digestive peristalsis and is conducive to bowel health. Brush up to the chest and neck and over the shoulders, up the arms and reach as much of the back as you can, continuing firmly but gently to brush and stimulate the skin.

If areas are particularly swollen or sensitive, due to arthritis, then avoid direct brushing over these. If restriction of movement is such as to make the procedures difficult, then a family member or friend can do this for you.

Ideally skin brushing should be followed by a shower or a bath. The tingling sense of well-being which will be felt is worth the effort. The benefits to the arthritic are of speedier elimination of acid wastes and a far healthier degree of internal drainage. It is suggested that this be done five or six days a week, or every day for three weeks, and then leaving a week free. The break somehow allows the degree of response to remain high, whereas constant use eventually produces a slowing down of this desirable reaction.

Shock absorbers in the shoes

The use of shock absorbing insoles in shoes has been proved to produce up to 50 per cent reduction in pain and stiffness in people suffering with arthritic changes in the pelvis and low back by the simple means of reducing the stress passing through these regions. It is suggested therefore that anyone thus afflicted should ensure cushioned soles or insoles. One simple method is to buy jogging shoes which are superbly cushioned and to use these for everyday walking around the home and garden. A good shoe shop will advise on alternative methods of improving cushioning in shoes.

We have considered general body mechanics and exercise, as well as relaxation methods in the relief of pain and stiffness. We have also looked at some safe methods of hydrotherapy, at ways of using muscle energy and pressure, and at chilling and stretching methods. Obviously, these methods all deal with existing states of dysfunction in joints, and so presume a degree of existing stiffness and disability. In order to reverse the potential worsening of this condition it is also vital that we consider the biochemistry of the body. This means that we must consider nutrition in our search for safe self-help methods.

4.

Arthritis and Nutrition

Probably no aspect of life has such a dramatic influence on health generally, and on arthritis (in all its forms) in particular, as what we eat. There are a number of specific nutrients which, when in short supply, have been found to influence arthritis adversely. These can greatly assist in checking and sometimes overcoming the symptoms of arthritis. Additionally, there are foods which irritate and aggravate arthritis. These can include either highly acidic foods, or foods to which the invididual is 'sensitive', or allergic.

Deficiencies
We are all genetically unique and this has been shown to result in individuals having idiosyncratic requirements for particular nutrients. Certain people need far more of some particular nutrients than others, and this requirement manifests itself in a particular

pattern of symptoms. The requirement may be for any of the nutrients (e.g., minerals, vitamins, amino acids) which the body requires for normal functioning. In regard to arthritis we would normally be concerned with a particular group of nutrients which is involved with the integrity of the ligaments, tendons, cartilaginous tissue, muscles and bones. We will now examine each of these groups.

Minerals

Calcium

This is the mineral which is most useful for improving the tone and elasticity of the soft tissues around the joints. Calcium also assists in transportation of nerve impulses, from one part of the body to another. This function is directly involved with another aspect of the work of calcium, which is in promoting the efficient contraction and relaxation of muscles. Normally, over 90 per cent of calcium which is ingested is incorporated into the body structures with the rest being involved in other functions, including those mentioned above. Surveys in the USA indicate that over 30 per cent of the population is calcium deficient. With inadequate calcium, muscles cannot contract adequately. This can lead to joint instability. Also, if calcium is lacking, there is a 'softening' of bone, which can lead to overprotective spasms in the soft tissues supporting these bones, with consequent stiffness and pain. In such circumstances, simply taking calcium is unlikely to be effective.

since it interacts with other nutrients making extra zinc and magnesium also necessary to correct calcium deficiency.

Magnesium

This nutrient is often called 'nature's tranquillizer'. It enhances the body's ability to contract muscles. The symptoms of magnesium deficiency include muscle tremors, as well as loss of calcium and potassium, leading to cramps. Since the processing of food often results in magnesium being eliminated, there is wide-spread deficiency in modern society. It is vital that calcium and magnesium are supplemented together, preferably in a ratio of two parts calcium to one part magnesium.

Manganese

This is a vital component of enzymes involved with the musculo-skeletal system. Manganese deficiency is evident when collagen (the supporting soft tissue material) is not functioning normally. It has been said by experts in physical therapy that supplementation of manganese doubles the success rate of the treatment of joint problems.

Zinc

This most important mineral is vitally linked with the healing of irritated tissues. It is also involved in calcium metabolism. In treating rheumatoid arthritis, Dr Carl Pfeiffer, of the famous Brain-Bio Center in America, has used zinc with great success. He points out that arthritic sufferers usually show a high copper level in the body. He believes that zinc drives copper from the inflamed joint. In clearing heavy metals from the body, when they are in excess, amino acids (parts of protein) have been combined with other nutritional methods. Thus, when copper is in excess and zinc is being used to counter this, the amino acid l-histidine has been successfully used in doses of between one and six grams a day to help normalize the biochemistry of the inflamed joints. Zinc is used at Pfeiffer's Center in doses of 200 mg a day, until improvement is noted (for up to twelve weeks). The only side effect noted was mild diarrhoea. Zinc also has a beneficial effect on the defence mechanism of the body. Vitamin B_6 is employed at the same time as zinc therapy, as both are closely associated in their work.

All minerals mentioned in this chapter are best taken as 'chelates'. This means that they are linked with easily absorbed proteins, which enables better uptake and utilization by the body.

Vitamins

Vitamin B complex
The vitamin B complex has special importance to the functioning of the nervous system. It is involved in the stability of nerve structures and function, as well as the musculo-skeletal system. Muscle tone is particularly influenced by vitamin B_1 (thiamin), which also helps in the

elimination of toxic wastes. Vitamin B_3 (niacin) has been shown to stimulate local circulation, improve joint mobility, decrease stiffness, and bring relief to many distorted and painful joints. Dr William Kauffman of Stratford, Connecticut, USA, first used B_3, in single one gram doses, for treating arthritis, and found it often helped. A trial in Sweden has also shown it to be effective, and also well-tolerated. Limitation of movement often responds dramatically to B_3. Vitamin B_5 (pantothenic acid or calcium pantothenate) has also been used to help the arthritic condition, by virtue of its effects on the adrenal gland, which defends us against stress. Many arthritic sufferers have been shown to be deficient in B_5.

Vitamin C

This vitamin takes part in many body processes. The health of bones, tendons, cartilages and connective tissues depends upon its presence in adequate amounts. Its major function from our viewpoint is that it is involved in the synthesis of collagen. This is a protein fibre found throughout the body's soft tissues, and is its main supporting tissue. It strengthens the 'cement' of the body giving it integrity and stability. When vitamin C is deficient all body tissues are affected. Muscles weaken, and ligaments grow so weak that they cannot support the joint.

Vitamin D

This is vital for the adequate uptake and utilization of calcium.

The above nutrients are the most critical ones of which the arthritic sufferer should be aware. It is of course possible to obtain all these from a well-balanced diet, such as the one outlined later in this chapter. However, modern farming and processing methods may produce foods with insufficient of some these substances to quickly correct existing deficiencies. Therefore some short-term supplementation is often beneficial. The dosages suggested for these substances follow:

Calcium	1 g daily	Ideally as chelates or orotates.
Magnesium	0.5 g daily	
Manganese	50 mg daily	
Zinc	100–200 mg daily	

Vitamin B_6	50–250 mg daily
Vitamin B_1	100 mg daily
Vitamin B_3	0.5–1 g daily (as niacin*, not nicotinamide)
Vitamin B_5	250–750 mg daily
Vitamin C	1–3 g daily
Vitamin D	400 i u daily

* May cause short-term flushing.

These should be taken for at least three but preferably six months, before reviewing the situation; however, if symptoms are well under control then dosages should be stopped. (See end of chapter for suppliers of supplements.)

General rules of eating and diet
1. Digestion begins in the mouth. Food should be eaten slowly and chewed thoroughly.

2. Avoid foods that are very hot or very cold.
3. Avoid drinking any liquid with meals as this interferes with digestion (as does any liquid taken up to an hour after a main meal).
4. Prefer simple meals as these are easier to digest than those with sauces. Avoid combinations of certain food that produce indigestion, such as protein and carbohydrate (e.g., bread and cheese, or fish and chips).
5. Avoid fried and roasted foods as these are difficult to digest.

In any rheumatic condition the following pattern of diet will lead to an overall reduction in pain and improved function, especially if accompanied by the other methods outlined in this book. As individual differences exist it is difficult to be specific about desirable eating patterns. Therefore the following suggestions focus on those foods which should be avoided.

Salt and salted food: Avoid completely and replace with moderate use of potassium chloride and herbs.

Meat: Use modest amounts of fish or free range poultry, i.e., no more than three ounces daily. In acute conditions this should also be abandoned in favour of vegetable protein (pulse and cereal combinations).

Dairy produce: Apart from a little (four ounces daily) live goatsmilk yogurt, replace

milk with soya milk, and cheese with tofu
(soya curd).

White flour or white rice products: Replace
with wholemeal, millet and brown rice.

Sugar: Avoid completely.

Tea, coffee, chocolate, cola drinks: Avoid,
replacing them with herb teas, dandelion
coffee and fresh vegetable drinks, or yeast
extracts (if low salt), or spring water.

*Processed, pickled, smoked, preserved, tinned
foods*: Avoid vinegar, pepper, curry.

Frozen foods: Strictly limit these, especially
commercially frozen foods.

Acid fruit: Strictly limit plums, berries, citrus,
etc.

The diet should comprise at least 50% raw
food in the form of vegetables, sprouted seeds
(leave these out of your diet if you have
rheumatoid arthritis), seeds, nuts, wholegrains
and some fruit. Breakfast should be seed
(sunflower, pumpkin, linseed, etc), nut, grain
millet or oat flakes mixed together with some
fresh or dried non-acid fruit. In sub-acute
conditions a little live yogurt can be added. One
main meal each day should be a mixed salad
with seeds and wholemeal bread, a rice savoury
or a jacket potato. For five days of the week,

the other main meal should be a cooked vegetable meal with a protein savoury (either fish or chicken or ideally a combined cereal and pulse dish). On the other two days a second salad meal should be eaten. Drinks should be as indicated above.

This diet is designed to minimize the chances of a continued deficiency; as well, it should reduce the acidification and toxification of the body, which is so prevalent a factor in arthritic and rheumatic conditions. By combining the suggested supplementary intake with this diet the self-healing mechanisms of the body will be given the best possible chance to carry out their task of repair to damaged areas and organs.

Fasting

Fasting is useful in the body's detoxification. It is one of the oldest methods of healing. It is instinctive in sick animals and probably was in primitive men, too. As well as having psychic and spiritual benefits, fasting can be useful in preventing disease, if carried out sensibly. It is often confused with starvation but, strictly, it is abstinence for a given time from solid food, and not from liquids. The last point is controversial. Some experts say fasting is most effective if only water is taken, whereas others, myself included, advocate the intake of fruit and vegetable juices. Some strange things may happen to the body during a fast and it is best to understand them before beginning one so that they do not cause anxiety; they are, after all, signs of rejuvenation.

Fasting often results in a furred tongue, 'sick' headache, bad breath, dark and often offensive urine, and sometimes unusual bowel movements. The degree and intensity of these signs of detoxification will vary greatly from person to person, often depending on the underlying health and vitality of the individual, as well as on the type of fast being used. Surprisingly, hunger is often not noticed after the first day.

Fasting can be seen as the preparation for self-healing. It is not a cure for anything. It provides a chance to eliminate toxins which are preventing the body from healing itself. So it is important not to treat the initial signs of fasting, such as a 'sick' headache, with any drugs or potions that will suppress them. The initial discomforts will soon disappear. A short fast may not be long enough for all these things to happen, but by repetition, the intensity of the symptoms of the first fast will diminish. In time, fasts may be enjoyed without marked symptoms, which is a sign of increased health.

If a chronic illness is involved, such as arthritis or an allergic or catarrhal condition, then there is a good case for daily enemas or, for those who prefer, a herbal laxative, before and after the fast. Breaking the fast correctly is also important. After any length of time without solid food there must be a gentle transition back to a full diet. It is also important that during a fast some exercise is taken; staying in bed is seldom necessary, but plenty of rest is. Therefore it is unwise to fast while carrying on normal work. It is also unwise to drive during a fast because dizziness may occur. Fresh air and rest are important as is the avoidance of stress. This explains the popularity of health farms and hydros, which offer a restful environment.

Three-day fasts, done over a weekend, are a good introduction and such a fast is set out below. A three day detoxification, every four to six weeks, over six or twelve months, will produce a dramatic improvement in health. Alternatively you might prefer to fast for one day each week. A light meal can be eaten midday on a Saturday, followed by juice on Saturday evening through to Sunday evening, with the fast being broken Sunday evening or Monday morning. Such a fast, lasting twenty-four to thirty six hours every week or fortnight will also be beneficial to health.

In all cases, the aim of fasting is to rest the body from the constant onslaught of food. This principle can also be applied to everyday eating to make us feel more vital and lively. For instance 'breakfast' implies that we have been for a period without food. This is true if the last meal of the day was at 6 p.m. and breakfast is at 7 a.m. or 8 a.m. But if we eat after nine then the digestive system will barely have finished coping with the evening meal before the next lot of food starts to arrive. Such a pattern of eating makes people sluggish and lethargic. By eating earlier in the evening, with no snacks later on, you can be livelier in the morning and have a rested digestive system, ready for the next day. Longer fasts should only be undertaken with the help of a qualified nutritionist.

Preparing for a fast
The day before fasting, a herbal laxative such as
psyllium seeds, or a broth made of flax seeds
(linseed), or castor oil, should be taken after the
midday meal, which should itself be light
(vegetarian for preference, such as a mixed
salad or a vegetable soup). In the evening have a
light fruit meal (pear, apple, grapes), or a
vegetable broth (recipe follows). On rising the
next day drink either camomile or peppermint
tea (unsweetened), a cup of vegetable broth,
half a cup of spring water with half a cup of
carrot juice, or warm or cold apple juice (diluted
with water). A selection of one of these items,
or bottled spring water, should be consumed at
two to three hour intervals during the day,
making sure that vegetable broth is consumed
at least twice during the day (not less than one
pint daily), and that the total daily liquid intake
is not less than $2\frac{1}{2}$ pints, and not more than 4
pints. If fresh vegetable juice is not obtainable,
then Biotta vegetable juice is available at most
health food stores, and is suitable for fasting as
it contains no preservatives, other than lactic
acid, and is guaranteed organically grown.
Carrot and beetroot are the ideal juices.

Continue this pattern for the two or three
days of the fast and finish on the evening of the
final day by eating one of the following 'meals':
puréed cooked apple or pear; puréed carrot, plus
a little puréed vegetable soup; live, natural
yogurt can be eaten with either of these
choices. All food should be thoroughly and
slowly masticated. The next morning eat yogurt

and grated apple or fresh pear, and have a salad and jacket potato for lunch, continuing with a normal pattern of eating. (Processed foods, such as white flour and sugar products, should be avoided and the diet should consist of wholefood). If any of the above foods cause allergies they should, of course, be avoided. For this reason it is best to fast under some degree of supervision.

If possible, a herbal laxative or castor oil or a warm water enema should be used on the last evening of the fast. If the patient is chronically ill, then daily small water enemas should be used during the fast. Half a pint of water at body heat is recommended.

The hygiene of the bowel can be further improved by employing one or all of the following, both during the fast and for a week or so afterwards. Take a quarter teaspoonful of Vital-Dophilus or half a teaspoonful of Super-Dophilus daily. These highly concentrated acidophilus products will enhance the flora of the bowel while the Vital-Dophilus is suitable for people who are milk sensitive. Also, stir a teaspoonful of fine green clay powder into a small glass of spring water and allow it to settle for an hour. Drink the water, but not the sediment. The clay has a detoxifying effect and soothes the bowel. (See end of chapter for list of suppliers.)

During the fast
Expect to feel lethargic during the fast, and perhaps a degree colder than usual so wear an

extra layer of clothing. Rest as much as possible since the aim is to allow energy to be employed towards healing, not diffused in unnecessary activity. Take no medication of any sort. In people of normal weight the fast will result in a number of predictable and beneficial effects, but it will not have the same physiological effects in very overweight individuals. One of these beneficial effects is the release of a growth hormone by the pituitary gland. This hormone has many functions including fat mobilization. As individuals of normal weight release more of the hormone than overweight ones the benefits are greater for them. A short fast by an overweight person is quite in order, provided that their general health is stable (and they do not suffer from diabetes, etc). Fasting is safe if employed correctly, and is one the swiftest detoxifying and health-promoting methods available. Try it regularly.

Make your own vegetable broth

If possible use organically grown vegetables. If this is not possible then scrub vegetables well before use. Into 4 pints of spring water place 4 cupfuls of finely chopped beetroots, carrots, thick potato peelings, parsley, courgette, and leaves of beetroot or parsnip. Use no sulphur-rich vegetables, such as cabbage or onions, which might produce gas. Simmer for five minutes over a low flame, to allow the breakdown of vegetable fibre and the release of nutrients into the liquid. Cool and strain, using only the liquid and not the leftover vegetable content. Do not add salt, as this broth will contain ample natural minerals and will provide nutrients without straining the digestive system. Also, it is alkaline and neutralizes any acidity resulting from the fast. Drink at least 1 pt of this nutritious broth daily during the fast.

Allergy

One of the most important contributions to our knowledge of arthritic conditions has come from practitioners dealing with allergies. Many of these practitioners call themselves clinical ecologists, and they have shown that by the removal from the diet of foods which cause allergies, many arthritic conditions can be improved. In attempting to ascertain which foods produce allergies in patients, many practitioners use a period of fasting to clear the body of all toxic substances. They then reintroduce foods one at a time to gauge the body's reaction. In this way they can build a picture of undesirable foods which should be avoided. Sometimes, those foods which cause a reaction can be reallowed by using a rotation diet. The allergy-producing foods may be consumed on infrequent occasions, say once a week. By eliminating dairy produce and refined carbohydrates (e.g., white flour and sugar) from the diet, we remove some of the foods which most commonly cause allergies.

By employing short and regular fasts, and by using nutritional supplements, the likelihood is that food sensitivities or allergies will be further eliminated. However, it may be that a commonly

eaten food continues to irritate the joints and
this may show up after a fast when the
particular food is reintroduced. If such a food is
identified, then it should be used sparingly in
the diet. It is also useful to identify other foods
belonging to the same group as the one which
causes the allergy. These should also be rotated,
so that they are not used more than once in five
days.

In general, a combination of all the factors
discussed above, namely diet, detoxification and
replenishment of deficient nutrients, provides a
framework for alleviating arthritic conditions of
all sorts. In addition, exercise and hydrotherapy
are beneficial.

Suppliers

Vital-Dophilus is available from Klaire Laboratories,
126 Acomb Rd, Acomb, York YO2 4EY

Super-Dophilus is available from G & G supplies, 175
London Road, East Grinstead, Sussex.

Chelated minerals, Green Clay and vitamins are
available from Larkhall Laboratories, 225 Putney
Bridge Rd., London SW15 2PY.

5.

Rheumatoid Arthritis

The causes of rheumatoid arthritis are not fully understood. Although the minutia of the actual changes involved in the arthritic process are well documented, the causes remain largely a matter for speculation. One cause which applies in some cases only, involves the presence in the arthritic joint of virus particles. This has led to a line of enquiry which points to some common childhood ailments as being a possible starting point, and also to immunization against these conditions being implicated.

Rubella vaccination and juvenile (and adult) arthritis
One condition in particular has a history of producing juvenile arthritis and that is Rubella (German Measles) and vaccination against this. German measles is not a particularly serious problem for children, but vaccination is performed in order to protect the female

population, so that they do not contract the disease when they are of childbearing age and thereby risk having malformed babies. Males are immunized in the hope that this will reduce the general level of the infection in society, in order ultimately to wipe it out.

All this is laudable in its intention, if debatable as to its efficacy. Unfortunately one of the commonest side-effects of rubella vaccination is arthritis and polyneuralgia. Much of this is transient and leaves no permanent damage. However there is evidence of wider damage in many young bodies.

How widespread is this?

The following report appeared in *Science* (26 March 1977): 'The HEW reported in 1970 that as much as 26 per cent of children (over 1 in 4) receiving rubella vaccination developed arthralgia or arthritis. Many had to seek medical attention, and some were hospitalised.'

Adults too are vaccinated against this, since young women who did not contract the illness in childhood, and who are anticipating parenthood might well be persuaded as to its desirability.

In Canada it is reported (Humanitarian Society, Quakertown, Pennsylvania 1983) that 30 per cent of adults given rubella vaccine suffered arthritis attacks within four weeks, some of these of crippling intensity. Dr Glenn Dettman of Australia reports that live rubella viruses have been found in one third of children and adults suffering rheumatoid arthritis.

As recently as October 1985, the New England

Journal of Medicine reported; 'Infection, or immunization with rubella virus, has been recognized as producing acute synovitis (inflammation of joint capsules) which although usually self-limiting has been reported to recur for months or years after the acute stage'. The report continues by stating that a full 35 per cent of people suffering chronic joint disease (such as juvenile rheumatoid arthritis, spondyloarthritis and polyarticular rheumatoid arthritis) were carrying rubella virus particles. These were *never* found in people who did not have joint diseases.

It is clear therefore that a large proportion of rheumatoid arthritis is, partly or totally, the result of immunization techniques. Another major cause of rheumatoid arthritis, which is partially understood, involves what is called autoimmune processes. This means that an allergic reaction is underway, and the tissues which are being reacted against, as being 'foreign' to the body, are its own joints and soft tissues. Thus the body is literally appearing to want to eliminate or destroy its own tissues. Being allergic to oneself is not a pleasant prospect, and understanding just how this might have occurred requires awareness of the immune system, the body's defence mechanisms and health.

One major aspect of immune function is related to the thymus gland which lies within the chest. The thymus is responsible for mobilizing the white blood cells of the body into action against any possible invading micro-organisms or foreign protein (cancer cells, malabsorbed foods, etc). The cells which it calls up in a crisis are called T-cells (T for thymus). These in turn produce substances called lymphokines which are natural defenders of the body (one of these is called interferon which is a potent anti-cancer weapon produced by the T-cells).

The T-cells also produce macrophages which literally 'eat up' or engulf bacteria, cancer cells, etc. Part of the T-cell function is to balance against the overzealous action of other defending white blood cells, called B-cells, which produce antibodies against any invading substances or bacteria. If there are too few T-cells, then the B-cells can be so active that they destroy the very tissues of the body. The T-cells are suppressors of over-enthusiastic B-cell function, and so the balance between these different 'soldiers' of the body is a vital part in maintaining health.

When autoimmune disease is operating, such as in rheumatoid arthritis, cancer, ulcerative colitis, multiple sclerosis and diabetes, B-cells are predominant, and T-cells in short supply. Part of any strategy to improve such a condition should therefore involve an attempt to rebalance this situation, and to assist thymus activity and consequent T-cell activity. The mineral and vitamin support, recommended in this and previous chapters, will enhance T-cell function considerably. The nutrients most valuable in this task are also strong antioxidants (see below) which makes them doubly useful. They include vitamins C and E, as well as a number of the B complex vitamins (notably B_6, B_5 [pantothenic acid] and folic acid) as well as zinc and selenium.

Free radicals and arthritis

When metal is exposed to oxygen for too long it oxidises or rusts. When an apple or potato is peeled, it changes colour rapidly as it oxidises. When hair is bleached with hydrogen peroxide it changes colour as this powerful oxidant destroys the pigment (and something of the structure) of the hair. As we get older our tissues, such as skin, show signs of ageing, and wrinkling becomes apparent; this too is largely a process of oxidation.

All of these examples involve the presence of substances called free radical oxidisers, highly active elements which, because of their structure, are able to disrupt other cells, by 'stealing' atoms from them, which alters their structure. A wide variety of changes ensue and it is not within the scope of this book to fully explore these, apart from pointing to the fact that many inflammatory processes involve a virtually uncontrolled series of free radical chemical changes.

It is a part of the normal body defence mechanism to produce free radicals, a process by which blood cells destroy invading enemies. If the body produces its own free radical, and with it destroys an invading micro-organism, for example, then it relies upon the presence in the body of antioxidants, to 'quench' the process when it has usefully done its job.

There are, within the healthy body, a large number of free radical deactivators, or scavengers, which mop up surplus oxidative elements such as this, preventing tissue damage. If however there are excessive free radicals present (due to a diet rich in fats or sugars, cigarette smoke, alcohol, chemical pollution, etc) and inadequate antioxidant nutrients in the body (Vitamins A, C, E, B_6, selenium, etc) then the process can get out of hand and tissue damage may result. This process is now thought to be the starting point of many cancers (the free radicals can damage the genetic blueprint of the cell, the DNA, thus causing it to mutate) as well as the atheromatous changes in blood vessels which are the beginning of cardiovascular disease, and also of aspects of arthritis. Certainly in rheumatoid arthritis some of the inflammation involves free radical activity. Thus the same nutrients which enhance immune function are the ones which damp down excess free radical oxidation.

There have been attempts to find a dietary pattern which would limit such activity in arthritic conditions in general, and in rheumatoid arthritis in particular. One such diet involves the use of particular essential fatty acids, derived mainly from fish, but also found in plants.

EPA and arthritis

Some years ago an American, Doctor Dong, concluded after treating his own arthritic condition, that the approach which achieved the best results involved the elimination from the diet of dairy products and saturated fats. This was before knowledge of free radicals was widespread, and indicates that he had found, by trial and error, a method of reducing substances in the body which are readily oxidised, that is animal fats. The eating of proteins such as fish and chicken was encouraged, on Dr Dong's diet, as was the abundant use of vegetables.

This is a simplification of the diet which he recommended but is of interest, since a study published in 'The Lancet', in January 1985, indicates that by reducing saturated fats from the diet (ie no dairy products and red meat) as well as increasing the sources of polyunsaturated fats (vegetable origin) and a particular type of essential fatty acid found in fish there was a marked improvement in the condition of rheumatoid arthritics. The essential fatty acid which was used was eicosapentenoic acid (EPA for short) which is derived from cold water fish and is available in health food stores.

It was found in medical trials that the group of rheumatoid arthritic patients who followed this pattern achieved markedly less swollen painful joints and less morning stiffness (a characteristic of rheumatoid arthritis) than did the control group of patients who took a dummy supplement. It is important to realize that the improvements noted were not clearly evident until twelve weeks of following the diet. The researchers point out that: 'Changes in tissue lipids (fats) are not seen until six weeks after a change in diet'.

When the participants in the study were re-examined, some months after the trial, the group of patients who had had the EPA supplements had deteriorated rapidly (within two weeks of stopping the supplements) indicating that the programme needs to be continued indefinitely if progress is to be maintained. This is an important injunction for anyone with a long term arthritic condition. Once improvement is noted it is most unwise to abandon the pattern of diet and nutrients being followed, as a return of symptoms is likely.

These methods are seldom able to approach the true causes of the condition in rheumatoid arthritis which, as indicated, remain a mystery. They do however provide a strategy by which control can be achieved safely, in many cases.

EPA is available in capsules of around 300 mg and the dose suggested is of 1,800 mg daily (six capsules per day) divided into three doses. Red meat was allowed in the medical trials only twice per week, and then only if lean cuts were used with visible fat removed. Dr Dong however suggested that it be permanently abandoned. Chicken was allowed if the skin was avoided. Sausage, bacon and all lunch meats were banned, as was whole milk, cheese and saturated cooking oils (lard, butter, hydrogenated shortenings and margarine).

Anyone attempting this pattern should eat an abundance of vegetables and whole grain cereal products (see the paragraph below about grain sensitivity in rheumatoid arthritis), avoiding white flour products and all sugar if possible. Alcohol should be avoided.

Before considering a number of nutrients which are useful in rheumatoid (and often in osteo) arthritis, it is essential that we look briefly at the role of the bowel in the production and maintenance of inflammatory joint processes such as rheumatoid arthritis. These same factors would act as irritants in osteoarthritis in most cases.

Bowel health and arthritis

As indicated in earlier chapters the element of food sensitivity, or actual allergy, is often considered to be a part of the process of inflammation in arthritis. Such processes often involve what is called malabsorption, in which partially digested proteins are allowed to enter the blood stream from the bowel, due to changes in the bowel's structure and function, which may go back to infancy. It is found that in weaning from the breast there is often an intolerance to some of the early foods introduced, especially to cows milk. For a variety of reasons humans cannot always tolerate the milk of other species, and cows milk seems to be a particularly difficult food to cope with. Other early problem foods involve the eating of grains, which along with milk, are fairly recent additions to human diet. These were only introduced to human diet in any quantity within the last 10,000 years, and man's digestive capacity having spent some millions of years without these substances, has shown a particular reluctance to accept them, especially in infancy. They play a major part in allergies in general, and in food intolerance and malabsorption in particular. Many rheumatoid arthritics benefit from eliminating grains and dairy produce.

There are other elements to consider in thinking about bowel health. We have living within us billions of micro-organisms which are vital to our health. Most of these inhabit the intestinal regions and there, in return for accommodation and food which we provide, they perform useful services such as synthesizing certain vitamins and generally assisting in digestive function. The intestinal flora as it is called, changes with the type of diet we follow. One which is rich in fats and refined starches (sugars, white flour products, etc) can be shown to severely compromise the flora, in its normal functions, and health suffers as a consequence. Again free radical damage may be involved, and there is a likelihood of such a diet producing a degree of constipation. In such a condition undesirable breakdown products remain too long in the bowel and can irritate the lining and cause local changes. For these and other reasons malabsorption problems (intake into the bloodstream from the bowel of undigested or partially digested protein and other particles) often result, and these can relate to inflammatory processes such as rheumatoid arthritis. The intestinal flora may also be severely compromised by the use of antibiotics, which destroy large amounts of friendly bacteria along with whatever else it is being aimed at. A substance called serotonin is produced by the body when foods to which we are sensitive enter the system. This is involved in the inflammation within the joints of rheumatoid arthritis.

The type of diet recommended in this book will enhance bowel function and intestinal flora health automatically. This could be further enhanced by the use of acidophilus concentrates. These are some of the friendly bacteria, and repopulation of deficient colonies is possible by the judicious use of those acidophilus products, mentioned on page 65. By paying attention to the adequate presence in the body of antioxidants (vitamins A,C,E, selenium, etc) and ensuring desirable essential fatty acids such as EPA, as well as taking care of bowel health, there is a reasonable chance that we can control rheumatoid arthritis. All the methods outlined in the sections dealing with exercise, self massage, trigger point treatment and especially hydrotherapy, are also helpful for rheumatoid arthritis. The stress reduction methods and the use of positive thinking all add to the body's chance of coping with the problem, and none should be neglected.

Some other specific factors of value in all arthritic conditions, including osteo and rheumatoid arthritis, are outlined below. Firstly we should consider that remarkable nutrient antioxidant selenium.

Selenium and arthritis

The mineral element selenium is a truly remarkable substance, being of value in the protection of the heart, as an anti-cancer agent and of value in arthritis, as well as having numerous other benefits to offer. In 1980, Norwegian studies showed that in rheumatoid arthritis selenium levels in the body were low, and that this was reducing the efficiency of a protective enzyme in the body called glutathione peroxidase. Such patients benefit from selenium being added to their nutrient intake. In osteoarthritis it has also been shown that supplementation with selenium reduces pain to injured and damaged joints, especially when combined with other antioxidant supplements, such as vitamin A, C and E (there are a number of combinations of A,C,E and selenium available). The same benefits noted in humans are found in animals suffering from arthritic joints, when selenium and vitamin E (they act synergistically) are given. Selenium's major role is as part of this powerful team of antioxidants, and as an enhancer of vitamin E. Doses of 50 to 100 mg daily of selenium are suggested, together with vitamin E, in doses of between 400 and 1,000 iu daily.

Vitamins and arthritis

We have briefly discussed these in Chapter 3 and the notes in this chapter are meant to expand on those specifically involved in inflammatory conditions such as rheumatoid arthritis, although most are of value in osteoarthritis as well. Both vitamin B_6 (pyridoxine) and vitamin B_5 (panthothenic acid) have been shown to have beneficial effects on different types of rheumatic complaint.

B_6 is found to have the following effects; it decreases finger pain, as well as stiffness and numbness in the hand, shoulder, hip and knee areas and it helps to prevent night-time cramps. Doses suggested are between 50 and 250 mg daily.

Vitamin B_5 has been used successfully in both osteo and rheumatoid arthritis, in doses of 500 mg daily (as calcium pantothenate). One of its prime roles is in promoting the body's own production of cortisone from the adrenal glands. (see below).

Vitamin C and arthritis

This versatile nutrient is a major part of the substance collagen (rheumatoid arthritis is sometimes called collagen disease). Collagen is the substance which comprises cartilage, the major shock absorbing tissue in joints, which is destroyed in arthritis. Vitamin C together with minerals such as calcium and magnesium and the vitamins A and B_2, as well as amino acids such as proline, will help to rebuild damaged collagen.

Natural cortisone

These nutrients (mainly vitamins C and B_5) are important for the health of the adrenal glands which produce the body's own cortisone. Adrenal function is depressed in arthritis, and also is the major sufferer from stress of all sorts. Support with B_5 and vitamin C is therefore helpful in reducing its burden and in helping its normal functions, one of which is the production of hormones such as cortisone. The natural production of cortisone carries no side-effects, but its introduction as a drug does. As indicated on page 81 doses recommended for B_5 are between 250 and 750 mg daily, and vitamin C, one to three grams daily.

Bromelaine and cysteine
Whilst not strictly a nutrient, bromelaine is a remarkable extract of a common food, pineapple, although the form which is produced commercially of this remarkable enzyme is derived from the stem of the plant. It was first introduced in the late 1950s and it is reported to have a wide range of activities including aiding digestion, being a relaxer of smooth muscle and an inhibitor of blood aggregation (ie it keeps blood the right consistency) aiding in cancer prevention and being an enhancer of wound healing. Above all, from the arthritic's viewpoint, it has major anti-inflammatory benefits with virtually no side-effects.

Bromelaine is useful in all cases of tissue inflammation and this of course includes most arthritic conditions. Since it is virtually non-toxic, bromelaine may be used almost ad lib, unless there is any sensitivity or allergy to pineapples. It comes in doses of 200 mg and one or two such tablets may be taken three times daily to aid inflammatory processes. These should be taken away from meal times, or the enzyme will become involved in digesting the meal (it is a protein digesting enzyme). Its pain relieving benefits are the result of its reduction of local swelling and inflammation, and not of any direct pain-killing ability.

Its activity in the body is enhanced, and indeed activated, by the simultaneous taking of manganese (see page 55 or the detoxifying amino acid cysteine. One to three g of this should be taken daily for a month — together with vitamin B_6 and vitamin C. The ratio of cysteine to vitamin C should be one part cysteine to three parts C in order to obtain maximum benefit. Diabetics should not take cysteine, but in all other cases of chronic ill health, and rheumatoid arthritis in particular, it is recommended. After one month reduce to 2 g daily, and after a further month reduce to a maintenance dose of 1 g daily, always keeping the ratio with vitamin C of 1:3.

Histidine

In many cases of rheumatoid arthritis it is found that there is heavy metal toxicity, such as aluminium, cadmium, lead, etc. This in itself leads to free radical activity, as well as other harmful effects. An amino acid fraction of protein called histidine has been used in the USA, in doses of 6 g daily, to good effect in such cases of rheumatoid arthritis. Interestingly the Russians use this for their cosmonauts as a part of anti-radiation protection.

Amino acids are available from health stores, or from Larkhall Laboratories (address on p. 68).

6.

Herbal and Other Remedies

A number of substances, some herbal and some derived from marine organisms, have been found to alleviate the symptoms of the arthritic patient. Such products include extracts of New Zealand green lipped mussels and deep water sharks. Some of these have remarkable effects on the symptoms of pain and inflammation of arthritic patients. In discussing aids and comforts to the symptoms of arthritis it is essential to bear in mind that nothing that these substances do is capable of making the condition worse, as is the case with some pharmaceutical drugs. There is of course no harm in disguising symptoms, such as pain (unless the usefulness of pain to prevent the undesirable overuse of an inflamed or damaged joint is thus obliterated so that the joint is then overused and damage increased).

Currently the most potent and 'safe' pain-reducing agent is an amino acid called phenylalanine. This occurs usually in the l-form, but there is also a right-handed, or d-form. This reduces the degradation of the body's own pain killers, the endorphins, and thus helps in the easing of pain. The combination of d- and l-phenylalanine is known as DLPA, and is available from health food stores. By taking two 375mg tablets about half an hour prior to meals, three times a day, for several weeks, pain of most sorts will diminish to tolerable levels, or will disappear altogether. If after that period pain has not gone, then the dosage can be doubled for a further two weeks or so. If, in rare cases, there is still no improvement, then the method should be abandoned. In most cases there is improvement within a week, and at that point the tablets should be stopped, unless there is a recurrence (after some weeks or months). It must be remembered, however, that even if the pain goes, the underlying condition remains unaltered, and the joints should not be overused. Pain can also be alleviated by taking vitamin B_3 (niacin). One gram a day is the recommended dosage.

Many herbal substances can help in a variety of ways. One of the most potent of these is the African herb Herpagophytum procumbens, which is better known as the 'Devils claw'. This can be obtained as a tea or as a tablet, and in many cases provides a means of eliminating acidic wastes, thus improving the condition of an arthritic joint. Use of this, or any other herbal method, should be accompanied by the use of the detoxification diet, explained earlier. The herbs discussed below are also helpful.

Alfalfa contains vitamins, minerals, trace elements, eight digestive enzymes and eight essential amino acids. It therefore rebalances the glandular system as well as the blood. It is well known in the USA as an arthritis aid. Burdock root is another useful herb. It is one of the best blood purifiers, and helps break down cholesterol and calcium deposits, and neutralizes poisons. It is especially useful for reducing swelling in joints. Also useful is celery seed which is a strong diuretic and has a high mineral content. Its penetrating oils make it a powerful remedy for rheumatism.

Comfrey root contains the powerful healer allantoin, which helps to repair blood vessels and eases internal pains. It cleanses both the intestines and the blood. Another useful plant is kelp which promotes glandular health. It particularly helps the thyroid and adrenal glands. It concentrates the supply of vitamins, minerals and trace elements from the sea, and gives the body the chance to produce most of the enzymes necessary for the removal of rheumatic and arthritic deposits. Finally, sarsaparilla is useful as a blood cleanser, and is specific for rheumatism. It also helps with glandular balance through its supply of natural hormones.

All herbs mentioned are obtainable from health food stores or herbal shops. They can be used either individually or can be made up into mixtures by a qualified herbalist in order to promote the functions indicated in their descriptions.

In a number of trials, both green lipped mussel extract and squalene (an extract from deep water sharks) have been shown to be capable of relieving arthritic conditions, sometimes to a remarkable degree. These should be avoided by those who are sensitive to fish.

These self-help methods in treating arthritis offer relief, and short-term gains, but long term relief relies on the removal of the causes, whether they be physical, nutritional or emotional.

7.

Stress and Emotional Factors

It is now well established that many forms of ill-health are directly related to our habitual thought patterns. Our consistent thinking patterns create our experience of life, and this can directly affect the ways in which we become ill. We have already discussed some of the ways in which habitual posture, as well as inadequate exercise, may contribute towards joint problems. We are also aware of the possibility of doing something positive through our eating habits, to assist the body to cope better with the stress of life. In terms of our emotional and thinking patterns we need, if possible, to identify those areas which may be contributing to the overall dysfunction of the body. If we only knew what was underlying our problems, we could take action.

The work of Louise Hay in America has identified particular thought patterns that often precede, or accompany, arthritic conditions. Those that cause most general disturbance include a tendency to be over-critical of others, of oneself and of life in general. Emotional states which most frequently promote arthritis include bitterness, resentment, criticism and a general feeling of being unloved. Rheumatism is often accom-panied by feelings of resentment, chronic bitterness, a desire for revenge and a lack of love and affection. All of these emotions can be released from consciousness and, with practice, replaced by compassion, forgiveness and love.

We have to go beyond the merely physical to the mental causes of our states of health. Using the relaxation and guided imagery methods described earlier and inserting positive thought patterns such as, 'I have compassion for others, and for myself: I accept joyful feelings', we can begin to replace negative feelings. Whatever has gone before, must be put aside, and we must become aware of our potential for health and happiness and realize just how much this depends upon our attitudes. The concepts that are most helpful in replacing the worn, old, habitual, negative thoughts and images include the uplifting ones of love, peace and joy. Love of others and of self has enormous healing power. It dissolves anger, releases resentment, dissipates fear, and opens the way to health and harmony. Louise Hay writes the following as an example of the sort of positive affirmation of these ideas.

Deep at the centre of my being there is an infinite well of love. I now allow this to flow to the surface. It fills my heart, my body, my mind, my consciousness, my very being, and radiates out from me in all directions and returns to me multiplied. The more love I use and give, the more I have to give — the supply is endless. The use of love makes *me feel good*; it is an expression of my inner joy. I love myself, therefore I take loving care of my body. I lovingly feed it, and my body lovingly responds to me with vibrant health and energy. I love myself therefore I provide for myself a comfortable home, one that fills all my needs and is a pleasure to be in. I fill the rooms with the vibration of love so that all who enter, myself included, will feel this love and be nourished by it. I love myself, therefore I work at a job that I truly enjoy doing, one that uses my creative talents and abilities, working with and for people, that I love and that love me, and earning a good income. I love myself, therefore I behave and think in a loving way to all people, for I know that that which I give out returns to me multiplied. I only attract loving people in my world for they are a mirror of what I am. I love myself, therefore I forgive and totally release the past and all past experiences and I am free. I love myself, therefore I love totally in the now, experiencing each moment as good and knowing that my future is bright and joyous and secure, for I am a beloved child of the universe, and the universe lovingly takes care of me now and forever more. And so it is.

This is something which might be read and repeated many times, to help to cancel past thought patterns, and to replace these with a guiding principle and ideal.

In general terms the following aspects of daily

living could also be examined to see if lifestyle and behaviour are contributing negatively to current health problems.

1. Avoid working more than ten hours daily and ensure that you have at least one and a half days a week free of routine work. If at all possible, an annual holiday 'away from it all' is advisable.

2. During each day, have at least two relaxation or meditation periods. Time should be set aside morning and evening, or just prior to a meal.

3. Perform active physical exercise for at least ten minutes daily, or for twenty-minute periods four times each week.

4. Balance the diet and eliminate stress-inducing foods and drinks.

5. Try to move, talk and behave in a relaxed manner.

6. Seek advice about sexual or emotional problems that are nagging away at the back of your mind, or which are causing conscious anxiety.

7. If there are stress-inducing factors at work or home, which can be altered, then take concrete steps to eliminate these.

8. Cultivate a creative rather than a competitive hobby, e.g., painting, DIY, gardening.

9. Try to live in the present, avoiding undue reflection on past events or anticipating possible future ones.

10. Concentrate on whatever the current task is, always finishing one thing before starting another.

11. Avoid making deadlines or 'impossible' promises that could lead to stress. Take on only what you can happily cope with.

12. Learn to express feelings openly in a non-belligerent way and, in turn, learn to listen carefully to other people.

13. Accept personal responsibility for your life and health. Do not look outside yourself for causes or cures, apart from the objective guidance and practical advice available from a professional health practitioner.

14. Greet, smile at and respond towards people in the way that you would like to be treated.

15. Introduce negative ionization into the home or work place and ensure adequate exposure to full-spectrum light.

Some of the ideas that have been looked at can be used positively to assist in dealing with underlying emotional or attitudinal habits, which have become fixed. These in turn may affect our physical well-being. Thus, changes in thought may lead to changes in the body and so diminish the prevalence of arthritis in our society. Self-help begins with awareness, and with acceptance of oneself. From that point progress is possible, and indeed probable.

Index